Dental Analogies

A collection of descriptive dental analogies

based on ideas from practicing dentists

3rd Edition

INTRODUCTION

Success in any profession, dentistry included, depends on the development of many skills. These include clinical and technical, business and organizational, communicative skills, and others. A practicing dentist uses any number of these attributes every working day.

Clinical mastery comes as the result of an adequate professional education, both through dental schooling and post-graduate continuing education. Business and organizational skills, following a rather shallow introduction in dental school, are developed experientially and through continuing education. The communication skills, cited as among the most important, have traditionally been slighted. As such, the palette of resources from which to choose to better one's communication abilities is small. This book was written to affect, profoundly and favorably, the communication skills of the dentist and dental team members.

Few would argue the premise that dental treatment should never be delivered to a patient without that patient's willful consent. In proper legal, ethical, and moral considerations, that patient's informed consent

must be based on a thorough knowledge of the facts —
of the pluses and minuses of both treatment and non-
treatment.

Autonomy in dental care helps the patient realize dental
self-actualization according to particular needs and
desires. Unfortunately, some presenters are unable to
adequately introduce the necessary treatment plan in a
way that creates true desire by the patient. With often
only a single chance to make this presentation to a
patient, this miscommunication may cause the dentist
to miss out completely on the opportunity to provide
the appropriate care for that particular patient. Thus,
the importance of the treatment plan presentation
cannot be overemphasized.

The treatment plan presentation is simply an organized
presentation of dental needs and a plan or plans for
solutions to answer those needs. It is akin to a sales
presentation which, on its highest level, concentrates in
finding a particular need and filling that need. Sales
presentations can be about intangibles, like insurance,
or something more substantive, like the delivery of
dentistry. The selling of the item is simply the formal

process by which needs are determined, communicated to the client or patient, and filled.

Unfortunately, many dentists find the idea of selling "raw," to a degree. Nonetheless, the fact remains: practically every successful person in his or her chosen profession proposes a service, idea, or product believing it will make the client's life better. For example, the primary goals in healthcare are to properly provide for patient needs and to promote health and well-being.

To meet those ends, adequate patient education is mandatory. Deviation from properly presenting alternatives is especially disserving in healthcare situations. Certainly, failure in the ultimate goal of helping the patient achieve dental self-actualization through autonomy is a worse ill than any act of selling.

Dentistry well-deserves the accolades bestowed upon it for its successes in preventive care and attending to patient needs in a timely, cost-effective, and honorable manner. Now, more is being demanded of the dentist, both from within the medico-legal arena and from patients themselves. Most patients want to be involved in treatment planning and it is the dentist's responsibility to be certain that each patient understands the thinking behind the doctor's proposed treatments.

In order for informed consent to work, the patient must have a crystallized mental image about his or her problem(s) and the proposed solution(s). To do this, dentists traditionally use brochures, diagrams, and models to educate patients. Unless these teaching tools can be sent home with the patient, residual effects are short-lived. Even when they ARE provided to the patient, they can get lost and even destroyed.

More modern educational means, including multimedia and the use of the intraoral camera, can bring the patient to an even higher level of understanding. However, it still may not be any longer lasting than that achieved by using the aforementioned tangible means. In addition, calling to attention one's own periodontal disease or broken tooth via an intraoral camera and 42-inch LCD monitor does not automatically create a want for treatment within that patient; rather, if not properly managed it may embarrass or, even worse, sell the patient on the service without emphasizing its implicit value. Such a "sale" does little to serve the patient properly and may even condemn the "service" to imminent failure.

What is a better way?

Every day, throughout the world, there are many sales presentations that result in the acceptance of things valued at hundreds of thousands of dollars and more. Of course, these presentations occur outside dentistry. Still, they do happen and the purchase of the service or product being presented is often predicated on the acceptance of an idea alone. In the business world, it is called "*selling the sizzle, not the steak.*" It is what many dentists hope to do at every treatment plan presentation. Sadly, it often meets with failure. The more clearly the patient understands the need and the prescribed solution(s), the better the chance of case acceptance and post-treatment satisfaction for both the patient and the dentist.

The direct, one-to-one information transfer between the minds of the dentist and the patient is the preferred communication method in dentistry, operating on an almost ethereal plane. "Modern" time constraints, attributed to increased paperwork and the like, make every patient's visit and what is said at that visit even more valuable.

In order to "sell the sizzle, not the steak," exact information must be shared. When done properly, the patient leaves with an indelible, yet satisfying, mental image that may be all it takes, either now or later, to resell the patient on the need for the prescribed care.

A strong means of information transfer involves the use of metaphors or *analogies* to help the patient arrange his or her own thoughts for maximum result. Note this example about the power of the human mind:

> *A wanderer in the old days of Egypt came*
> *up on a young man who was forever*
> *looking for a fast and easy way to make*
> *more money. This young man had done*
> *well for himself and was now looking with*
> *even more fervor and greed. The wanderer*
> *made an offer to the lad. "I can sell this*
> *magic lamp and secret formula, only once,*
> *for 1000 gold coins and I guarantee that,*

together, they can turn sand into gold."
Naturally, the young man was interested.
"You guarantee the formula?" "Or your
money is returned." the wanderer
countered. The lad succumbed to the offer
and the deal was struck. "The only
condition that will make the formula not
work." added the wanderer as he handed
over the lamp and incantation, "is if, while
rubbing the lamp, you happen to think of a
monkey with a red tail. Then, the formula
will not work."

Woe is this young man who will now find it nearly impossible to not think of a red-tailed monkey.

So strong is the human communicative experience.

Most people cannot create and deliver such clever narratives as that scripted above. For them, a source of descriptive stories to help make points is needed. "Dental Analogies" is the first book of that kind. It is a collection of ingenious analogies created from hundreds of ideas from practicing dentists from across America and presented in a very useable format – including an expansive index. These dentists are using these analogies every day and report that they do, indeed, work – and work well.

As a reference, this book's analogies provide the dentist and team members many stories to share with patients that successfully compare various dental modalities to more familiar laymen's situations. Afterwards, the patient has a greater understanding of the dental condition.

Consider this example: A long-lost dental patient may question the need for comprehensive periodontal therapies like root planing and curettage, subgingival irrigation, and even surgery, citing the absence of significant symptoms. An analogy such as that found on pages 80-81 can be used. It compares the problem and its solutions to a failure to provide regular oil and filter changes for an automobile (with the concomitant expense and inconvenience of a major engine overhaul, et cetera.) Thus, the patient better understands why one brief dental "cleaning" cannot undo what years of neglect have caused. Additionally, it does not point a finger nor does it belittle the patient. It simply redirects the patient's mind to a more familiar problem that is better understood and accepted.

Julian Jaynes, in *The Origin of Consciousness in the Breakdown of the Bicameral Mind* (Houghton Mifflin, Co., Boston, 1976) wrote: "Understanding a thing is to arrive at a metaphor for that thing by substituting something more familiar to us. And *the feeling of familiarity is the feeling of understanding* (authors' emphasis)." A metaphor is a figure of speech in which a word or phrase literally denoting one kind of object or idea is used in place of another, suggesting a likeness or analogy between them.

This book of analogies is helpful not just for answering questions and objections, but for anticipating them as well. For example, before presenting a case to a patient that involves implants or several units of crown and bridge, pages 92 through 114 could be referenced. From these the financial coordinator or the doctor could select analogies best-suited to the particulars of that patient's hobbies, occupation, and other interests. Maximum effectiveness is realized if the financial coordinator or doctor has really gotten to know the patient personally.

One of dentistry's most respected figures, Dr. Lindsey Pankey, once said, "*Never treat a stranger.*" He proposed up to 22 separate questions that can be used to get to know a patient before initiating treatment (*A Philosophy of the Practice of Dentistry*, by Lindsey D. Pankey and William J. Davis, Medical College Press, Toledo, OH, 1987) Information like this can be used to help select the most appropriate analogies for a treatment plan presentation.

Some dentists have integrated a study of these analogies in their team meetings and "huddles" – like an Analogy of the Day. One doctor reports excellent results educating his staff this way.

Readers may find it helpful to first review all of the analogies, noting the topics, keywords, and the layout. The extensive index in the back makes retrieval of an appropriate analogy quick and easy. The analogies should be modified and adapted to particular styles of practice and speech.

As new analogies are created, born from the many ideas that these will no doubt trigger, they can be written out on the available blank areas found throughout on the book's pages. In addition, we appreciate them being shared with us for future editions of *Dental Analogies*.

Please list The Topic, The Situation, The Patient's Question, The Response Using an Analogy, and Some Keywords. Email it all to drh20s@gmail.com or mail it to Dr. Rick Waters, 385 Pinewood Circle, Athens, GA 30606

We especially appreciate analogies that address the use of the LASER, implants, 3D x-ray, and other emerging dental technologies. Sharing your ideas with us eventually helps the entire dental profession, which is an implicit part of being in any profession. Most Dental Codes of Ethics state something to the effect that, "*The dentist has the obligation of making the fruits of his discoveries available to all when they are useful in safeguarding or promoting the health of the public.*" Such is how it should be. Thankfully, we have found that this is how it is.

We want to thank everyone who contributed ideas toward this book, especially Doctors:

W. Adams, G. Alex, D. Alleman, W. Allen, A. Allgood, T. Aspes, M. Babcock, R. Berlin, M. Binns, P. Bracken, S. Brewer, L. Broadrick, D. Brockington, B. Brooks, T. Brooks, C. Burch, W. Callahan, D. Cassidy, S. Cohen, A. Collins. T. Conner, C. Creager, L. Darby III, E. Douglas, R. Dyer, J. Elliott, S. Erwin, D. Felker, M. Gobbel, G. Goldstein, J. Harden, P. Hauser, M. Healey, K. Henry, K. Houston, R. Johnson. K. Kay. V. Koehler, L. Landers, H. Lanier Jr., J. Linatoc, J. Linuter, C. Little, G. Madray, R. Manus, C. Martin, F. Matthews, K. Mattison, T. McDougal, H. McLaughlin Jr., D. Mentz, B. Patrick, R. Piede, T. Pierce, B. Powell, S. Powell, S. Prince, N. Pylant, H. Rackley, J. Ralston, V. Riccardi, E. Salley, P. Salter, A. Sanchez, P. Shaw, S. Smith, S. Stein, S. Taylor. R. Wand, R. Waters. R. Waugh Jr., M. Webster, R. Weinman. K. White, E. Willis Jr., and M. Winter.

THE ANALOGIES

"COMPREHENSIVE EXAMINATION'

Situation: This patient is in a hurry and wants only the problematic tooth restored. She has no interest in comprehensive dental diagnosis and care at this time.

Patient: "Doctor, I really don't want to spend time and money on x- rays now. I just want this broken tooth fixed."

Response: "I understand your concerns, Sallie, and I assure you we will take care of you. But, we need a complete exam and x-rays to make absolutely certain that it is, indeed, the broken tooth causing your pain. The examination process helps me treat you properly. It's like sewing. When you make a dress, you cut and fit the pattern before committing yourself to the stitching. Since we have time and you are here, why don't we go ahead and determine all your needs?"

Keywords: sewing, time, expense

"COMPREHENSIVE EXAMINATION"

Situation: This patient wants his work phased or staggered, and doesn't want a complete examination, with x-rays, models, etc. He prefers his money be spent actually repairing his teeth, rather than for "extravagant items," as he views them.

Patient: "Doctor, I want to spend my money fixing my teeth, not for models and such. Just start fixing what needs fixing and after a while we'll have them all caught up, won't we?"

Response: "Well, Tony, we could do that. But I would like for us to still be friends outside the office! Let me compare it to automobile repairs. If a body shop repaired the outside of an accident-damaged car, neglecting to check internal parts like the radiator, there's a chance of later failure, causing the driver to maybe become stranded. The x-rays and models give us everything we need to make sure you are attended to properly. The little extra expense up front can actually save you a lot of money later in unplanned extra dental needs. With your permission, I'd like to begin the comprehensive exam today."

Keywords: comprehensive, examination, automobile, money, x-rays, diagnostic

"COMPREHENSIVE EXAMINATION"

Situation: This patient wants his treatment to be phased or staggered, and is not, at this point, interested in a comprehensive examination with x-rays, study models, etc. He prefers that his money be spent "fixing them, not for just looking at them," as he puts it.

Patient: "Doctor, I'd rather spend my money fixing these teeth than making molds and x-rays and such. Just start fixing them and after a few visits, they'll be caught up, won't they?"

Response: "Mr. Kennedy, we could do that. But then, I want you to still like me when we meet outside the office. If I were a contractor, building you a house, you and I would both insist on plans for the floor layout, the site elevations, the wiring plan, the heating and air plans, the cabinetry plans, etc. Can you imagine the differences in the house you would imagine and mentally plan and the one I would build without any plans? We would be redoing a lot of work. The only way I can properly begin to treat your dental condition is with plans, so we both know where we are heading.

That actually saves you money, since it eliminates redoing things at your expense. Plus, it minimizes surprises and the potential for extra expenses that we didn't count on."

Keywords: contractor, plans, comprehensive care, work-up, saves money, re-treating, treatment plans

"COMPREHENSIVE EXAMINATION"

Situation: This patient has come to the office needing teeth restored and figures to make the most of this visit. Gross calculus is evident and he is resistant to its removal, pre-restorative.

Patient: "Doctor, I don't want my teeth cleaned right now. Just fix the one that's broken. And, while you're in there, if you see any others that need fillings, go ahead and take care of them too."

Response: "Mr. Davison, you have calculus all over your teeth. And, there are others that need repair. But, it will take more time than this one visit allows. If I were an auto mechanic who allocated only enough time to rebuild a four-cylinder motor and in rolled a V-8, you know I'd be thrown off. The lack of parts and adequate time would pose serious problems. I am prepared to take care of your immediate problem today — the broken tooth that is sensitive. Before we do any more treatments, however, we must get your teeth and gums caught back up to health. As an example, if you wanted me to paint your rusty car, you'd want the rust stopped first, wouldn't you?"

Keywords: restorative, cleaning, painting, rust, limited treatment, engine overhaul, mechanic

"COMPREHENSIVE CARE'

Situation: This young lady only wants her teeth "cleaned" and is not currently interested in comprehensive dental care.

Patient: "I don't want a complete examination. I just want my teeth cleaned, that's all. I don't think anything's wrong since they don't hurt."

Response: "Ellen, if you became pregnant, you wouldn't just wait until delivery day to see the doctor, would you? You would become involved in proper prenatal care and then in follow-up care for the baby. That's known as comprehensive care. In dentistry, proper treatment involves the same thing, comprehensive care. Without that, your visit with the dental hygienist for a cleaning is partially wasted."

Keywords: pregnancy, comprehensive care

"COMPREHENSIVE CARE"

Situation: This gentleman acts disinterested in oral rehabilitation.

Patient: "I'd just as soon have you take the ones out that will cost a lot to fix and fill the ones that can be saved."

Response: "Mr. Williams, if I sent you on a late-in-the-day errand into a bad area of the city in a car with major engine trouble, you would be hesitant at best; and, when beginning a vacation, if your airline pilot told you that only two of the four engines work, but it will just make the trip take longer, you probably would worry a little. Trying to function with too-few teeth is just as risky. The jaw joints, muscles, and teeth's roots, are all susceptible to major trauma by carrying too heavy of a load. Then, when they fail, it is usually irreparable."

Keywords: fees, comprehensive care, airliner, engine failure, inner-city

"COMPREHENSIVE CARE"

Situation: The patient is receptive to major rehabilitative care, but would like to stagger the treatment over a longer time frame and wants to manipulate insurance benefits to maximize usage.

Patient: "Well, I guess if I need crowns, I need crowns. Let's do them one at a time and then, maybe halfway through, go ahead and start the partial so I can budget my money and will not have to withdraw my savings. Also, I'll be able to use up all of my dental insurance."

Response: "I appreciate your concern. I assure you we'll work with you every way possible that we can. I don't know if you have ever had to have your car's engine rebuilt, but you know that the mechanic would want to service and replace all of the parts at once so they would properly 'mesh,' so to speak. Your dental care must be provided in the same way – a precise and planned manner, for it to best succeed.

If your car's engine was restored bit by bit, you would end up with a jalopy and not a well-tuned, fine machine."

Keywords: accept, major treatment, time, phasing treatment, mechanic, engine overhaul

"COMPREHENSIVE CARE"

Situation: This young lady is eager to have bleaching and cosmetic care performed, but is not interested in correcting her restorative needs first.

Patient: "I would rather get my teeth looking pretty first. Then, we can do all of those fillings you talked about."

Response: "Ms. Pless. Certain sequences must be followed for cosmetic dentistry to work. It is similar to counted cross stitching. The fabric must be exactly perforated for the intended image to appear. Otherwise, the results would not be satisfactory. I know how badly you want a beautiful smile and the only insurance of a favorable result is proper attention to the details and your cooperation; I am ready to do my part if you are ready to do yours."

Keywords: cosmetics, cross stitch, sequencing care

"COMPREHENSIVE CARE"

Situation: This patient resists needed comprehensive care. Of several hobbies, one involves traveling.

Patient: "Doctor, I just don't see the need for that 'Cadillac' dentistry. Just patch me up for now and I'll be on my way."

Response: "Mr. Post. I wish it were possible to just 'patch you up.' Unfortunately, I think you are past that point. What I recommend, dentally, is much like crossing the ocean; you can't go just halfway and get there. You can fly on a jet airliner, take a freighter, or start off by rowing a boat. All of them might get you there eventually, but you would want to go with the sure thing. The treatment I propose is what I feel is in your own best interest for your comfort, function, health and appearance."

Keywords: comprehensive care, travel, rowboat

"COMPREHENSIVE CARE"

Situation: This patient has asked that you "patch her teeth up" for now.

Patient:"Doctor, can't you just patch up those fillings for now. When the teeth really need the crowns and all, we can do those then."

Response: "Mrs. Smith, you can imagine how tedious it would be to have to repair your family's clothes. Well, that is like the dilemma facing me today. I cannot in good conscience continue to patch your teeth. They must be rebuilt. There really is no other alternative."

Keywords: patching, socks, crowns

"COMPREHENSIVE CARE"

Situation: A patient wants his teeth "patched up" for now, indicating a desire for definitive treatments later.

Patient:"I do want to save my teeth. Can you patch them for now? I will have dental insurance next year and will be able to get everything fixed right, then."

Response: "Mr. Sprague, we can put you in a 'hold' state where we stop the disease process and monitor you very closely. Your dental needs can be likened to resurfacing highways. When too many potholes have formed, patching is no longer possible. Complete resurfacing is the only permanent solution. Please keep in mind that your needs cannot permanently be met with temporary fillings. If you are willing to take the risks of the 'hold' state, I will give in. But you must stay with us with regular visits in the meantime."

Keywords: 'hold' pattern, patching, resurfacing

"COMPREHENSIVE CARE"

Situation: This woman is intent on having "non-essential" back teeth removed, in lieu of repairing them.

Patient: "Doctor, you won't be able to see where those teeth were if you remove them, will you? They are the backmost two. I'll still have the other side to chew on."

Response: "Mrs. Nash, one of the functions of the teeth is support, meaning support of the face. When the fabric on a pillow is stretch tightly over the foam within, the pillow is pretty and inviting. If the foam had a piece torn off before being covered, the pillow would be unsightly. Your teeth support your cheeks and lips, preventing their collapse and excessive wrinkling. I want to do everything I can to help keep you happy and looking young."

Keywords: extraction, pillows, facial support

"COMPREHENSIVE EXAMINATION"

Situation: This patient questions the need for a comprehensive examination.

Patient: "Doctor, I really don't care to have all that examining done. Just fix this tooth that is bothering me."

Response: "Mr. Rogers, I understand your concern for that tooth and I can assure you we will take care of it. But, in order for me to restore it properly, I need to detect exactly what needs to be done. It is like a carpenter told me once: you should measure twice and cut once. An examination is the 'measure' that I need to do before treating you."

Keywords: examination, carpenter, measure, comprehensive examination

"X-RAYS"

Situation: This patient is adamantly against having radiographs made. They are necessary to assess the extent of decay prior to excavation and restoration.

Patient: "I don't like x-rays. My other dentist didn't bother with them. I just want you to fix that tooth, that's all."

Response: "Mrs. Trent, the x-ray I need is like a miniature blueprint. I need to know what will be left anchoring the rest-oration or crown, like blueprints show the foundation for a house. Without an x-ray, I cannot be sure of where the nerve is relative to where we are working, and I know you want to minimize the need for possible added expenses for things such as a root canal."

Keywords: x-ray, refusal, blueprint

"X-RAYS"

Situation: The patient is not interested in radiographs and is suspicious of the need for them.

Patient: "I don't want any x-rays taken unless they are absolutely necessary. Why do you need them in the first place if everything looks okay in my mouth?"

Response: "Mrs. Kelly, we only take 'necessary' x-rays. They are a lot like baby pictures; they can really help you appreciate changes! To tell if roots are resorbing and such, we have to have something to go back to for comparison. These initial radiographs help us do that."

Keywords: x-ray, necessary, baby pictures, baseline

"X-RAYS"

Situation: This patient is concerned about having radiographs made.

Patient: "I am really not crazy about having x-rays done. How many did you say? Sixteen? Can't you just fix what you see needs fixing? If it can't be seen, maybe it doesn't need fixing anyway!"

Response: "Mrs. Morgan, did you know that, over a period of time, frequent airplane flyers receive more x-rays than you'll get from these 20 films? That's just one of the reasons pilots are limited in the number of hours they can fly each month, since they can't line the planes with lead protection. You'll receive a very small dose since we use ultrafast film, a fast x-ray machine, and a lead apron. That sounds more attractive, doesn't it?"

Keywords: x-ray, flying, safety, airline pilot

"X-RAYS"

Situation: This patient is unconvinced of the need for a full radiographic series before the development of a comprehensive treatment plan.

Patient: "Doctor, with all of the recent talk about the dangers of radiation, I really don't want to have pictures made of all of my teeth. Can't you just x-ray the ones that look the worst and leave the others alone?"

Response: "I share your concern, Mrs. James. That's why we use an ultra-fast digital x-ray machine and lead aprons. You are safe. We need a complete survey of your teeth and gums much like an airline pilot uses radar to look all around her as she flies in clouds. We cannot see where we are going without x-rays, much like a pilot can't always see without radar."

Keywords: full mouth radiographic series, x-ray, radar, airline pilot

"PANORAL RADIOGRAPH"

Situation: This patient doesn't want a panoral radiograph made, justifying her decision based on already having had bite-wing radiographs made.

Patient: "I don't see why you can't get the information you need from the four x-rays you already took."

Response: "Mrs. Shaw, we can learn a lot from those bitewing films. They are like looking at photographs of individual trees in a forest. The panoral radiograph is like making a picture of the entire forest. It helps show us how the individual trees fit in."

Keywords: panoral radiograph, x-rays, forest, trees

"FEES"

Situation: This patient is quite a shopper, blindly eager for cheaper dentistry.

Patient: "Doctor, do whatever is cheapest. I won't notice the difference, since I never really look in there anyway!"

Response: "Mr. Bryant, selecting a type of dentistry just because it is the cheapest is like stopping a clock to save time or getting a haircut to lose weight. It really won't do you much good in the long run."

Keywords: fees, haircut, cheaper dentistry, clock

"FEES"

Situation: The patient questions the fee that you have presented him or her for comprehensive dental treatment.

Patient: "Doctor, that sure is a lot of money for just a little dental work, especially if it takes as few visits as you say."

Response: "I can appreciate your concern for the amount that you must invest. I would like to compare your dental rehabilitation to an artist's painting. The canvas, the oils, and the brushes might cost just $25.00 or so. It is the experience, skill, and knowledge of that artist transferring the $25.00 worth of materials into a priceless masterpiece in which you are really investing."

Keywords: fee, artist, painting, skill, masterpiece

"FEES"

Situation: This patient is looking for "cost-cutter" dental care.

Patient: "I don't want to spend any more than I have to. Just do the minimum necessary to get me by and I will get you to do the big stuff when it is necessary."

Response: "Mr. Moore... That would be like building a house and roofing it with just tar paper and no shingles. It might work for a while; but, you would have to call the roofer for the shingles when leaks started. By then, it might be too late. The extra expense of redoing damaged ceilings and wet insulation, not to mention the inconveniences involved, would be much worse than having invested in the shingles in the first place."

Keywords: roofing, shopper, expense, minimal care

"FEES"

Situation: This patient has been informed of the need for multi-hundred dollar care to save a tooth (endodontic therapy, buildup, crown, et cetera) and resents having to invest the money.

Patient: "Doctor, I can't see spending all of that money just to save this one tooth. I think it is just as well that you extract it."

Response: "Mr. Garner, just as a watch may stop if a gear loses one of its teeth, your bite will begin to be severely interrupted if you lose this tooth. If you were to have joint trouble in your hand, you wouldn't ask the doctor to cut your affected fingers off. Amputating your tooth is no different; just the thinking is. Our thoughts in the dental profession are to keep teeth whenever and wherever we can. As hand microsurgery has it costs, so does meticulous care for this tooth. But, I'll be the diagnostician, the radiologic technician, the radiologist, the anesthetist, the surgeon, and even the follow-up nurse. So, as you see the expense involved has really been kept in line."

Keywords: saving a tooth, expense, amputating finger, missing gear tooth, cost-effective

"FEES"

Situation: This patient has only a few teeth left and cannot understand why her dental prophylaxis fee is not less than if she had all of her teeth.

Patient: "My neighbor. Mrs. Allen, just had her teeth cleaned and the fee you charged her was the same as mine was today. I know she has almost all of her real teeth. What I can't understand is why my charge was the same when all you have to do is clean my bottom front six teeth that my partial is attached to."

Response: "Mrs. King, I can understand your wonder. It may seem that various fees are 'out of sync' at times. I think you'll understand from this analogy, though. If you were to enter a hospital for a tonsillectomy, the hospital's fee for that operating room is not much different from what it would be for a more complicated hysterectomy or other similarly involved surgery. The fee for today's dental visit is partially based on the infection control costs and supplies used, which are needed for everyone whether they have six or 32 teeth. (This can carefully be added to humor the patient who can be humored.) You wouldn't want me to reward you for having lost some of your teeth, would you?"

Keywords: prophylaxis, cleaning, fewer teeth, cheaper

"FEES"

Situation: This patient needs replacement dental prosthetic treatments, is concerned with fee increases, and is looking for discounts.

Patient: "The fee you quoted me for these dentures (or this bridge, et cetera) is three times what I paid for the originals 25 years ago! Why does dentistry cost so much more, especially since we are replacing old work. Isn't your job a little easier because it's already been done before?"

Response: "Mr. Jackson, dentistry can be compared to home construction. Remodeling a house is, in many ways, more involved than building a new one, especially when remodeling a fine home. Then, it can actually cost even more. Another example is that, compared to twenty-five years ago, new cars today cost roughly eight times as much. If dentistry has only gone up three-fold in that same period of time, could something really be wrong? Seriously, for something that serves you 24 hours a day, 7 days a week, and 52 weeks a year for who-knows-how-long, and even stays wet the whole time, it's a rather good investment, don't you think?"

Keywords: expense, relative to new-ear cost, replacement care, remodeling

"FEES"

Situation: This patient is looking for the least expensive alternative.

Patient: "Why does it always cost so much? Isn't there a cheaper way to fix my teeth?"

Response: "Yes. Mrs. Porter, just like there are different ways of building a house, there are various ways of restoring your teeth to health. With regard to houses, lots of different things go into it: the quality of materials, the skill of the builder, the camaraderie of the team, and others. If the costs ranged from $50 to $100 per square foot, no doubt the $50 per square foot resulted in some 'corners being cut,' so to speak. I want to make sure you understand and accept that we will have to do the same if we decide on an alternative treatment plan."

Keywords: alternative treatment plan, cutting corners, house, builder

"FEES"

Situation: This patient is cost-conscious, with the fee as the only criteria determining the treatment.

Patient: "Aren't dentures cheaper than crowns and bridges and root canals and all of that stuff?"

Response: "Yes, Mrs. Davis, they are. But so are wooden legs and wheelchairs and crutches compared to saving your legs. (The following can he added to the **Response** if the patient can be humored.) The cost of dying is less than continuing to live, but we don't use that to make the decision!"

Keywords: fees, dentures, leg prosthetics

"WARRANTIES"

Situation: This patient is in doubt about consenting to comprehensive dentistry, recently discovering that it should not be expected to last forever.

Patient: "Doctor, is what you are proposing to do for me going to last? My sister spent thousands of dollars on crowns and bridges twenty years ago and now she has to have hers all redone."

Response: "Mrs. Berryman, that is a good question that many people probably have been concerned with. Let me paint this picture for you. When you have a permanent done for your hair, you never really know what it'll be like the first time. But, you hope for the best. The hair's response to the chemicals and the way you treat your hair afterwards affect the perm. Still, the perm eventually grows out. With your teeth's history, it would be overly-optimistic to expect treatment to last forever. But, although we will give our absolute best here, as you will with your homecare, it may still have to be replaced many years down the road. At least there will be teeth on which to replace it."

Keywords: reconstructive dentistry, hair perm, longevity, do your best

"WARRANTIES"

Situation: This patient wants a warranty on his dental treatments.

Patient: "I go along with your ideas, Doctor, but if I am going to have to invest that much money, what kind of guarantee can you give me it will all hold up?"

Response: "Mr. Norton, life doesn't allow for guarantees. I provide all of my care as if it were for a family member each time. Let me share this with you. If your Maker's work wouldn't hold up in your mouth with any guarantees, you really can't expect me to give you a better guarantee than that, can you? However, if you do your best with your homecare as I will do my best delivering your dentistry, there's no reason to expect anything but the best."

Keywords: warranty, religion, guarantee

"DENTAL INSURANCE"

Situation: This patient does not understand the different levels of dental care delivery and fee tiers, and is upset at her insurance company's less-than-expected payment, which was based on a low UCR fee schedule.

Patient: "Why are your fees higher than what my insurance company says is 'usual and customary?' I had a dentist before who just let the insurance pay it all. Why can't you do that?"

Response: "Mrs. Farmer, your insurance coverage is between you and your insurance company. We have nothing to do with it. Our fees reflect the costs involved in properly treating you here. You know, jewelry can be stored in a cardboard box, but most people don't do that. An heirloom wedding dress could be put away for many years in a cardboard box, but people don't do that either. Fine dentistry demands precision that involves some expense. Many insurance companies prefer 'cardboard box'-type dental care, so to speak. I don't, and I'm sure you don't either. And, in the past, when your insurance 'paid it all,' either that doctor had extremely low expenses, he charged the insurance company a higher fee than usual, or you were part of a preferred dental provider organization. I hope it was the first."

Keywords: waive copayment, UCR, high fees, PPO, dental insurance

"PROCRASTINATION"

Situation: An elderly or middle-aged patient wants to spread her treatments out over several years, which would compromise proper delivery.

Patient: "Yes, Doctor, I understand what I need. But can't we spread it out over a few years to help with the bills. I can't handle all of it at once."

Response: "Mrs. Allen, I understand your dilemma. We will work with you every way we can. However, if your cardiologist diagnosed four blocked coronary arteries, you wouldn't expect him to treat just two now and repair the other two later. Thankfully, your dental problems are much, much less serious. But, we are affected by similar constraints. Proper care here means treating everything that needs it at the same time."

Keywords: coronary arteries, bypass surgery, comprehensive care, procrastination

"PROCRASTINATION"

Situation: Patient wants only the symptomatic problem taken care of and prefers to wait for others to appear before agreeing to definitive care or preventive action.

Patient: "I just want to have the tooth that's hurting fixed and when the others bother me. I'll let you fix them then."

Response: "Mr. Eaves, repairing that one tooth alone is like calling in a firefighter to put out a whole-house fire just in the kitchen area because that's where it started. You certainly would want your entire house and family's possessions saved. I think you will agree that those things are no more valuable than parts of your own body, which are truly irreplaceable."

Keywords: procrastination, fire, comprehensive care

"PERIODONTAL TREATMENT"

Situation: This patient is concerned about whether she is "off the hook" with respect to redeveloping periodontal disease, since she has now been through surgery to treat a previously-existing problem.

Patient: "Will I have to continue to worry about periodontal disease, even now, after my gum surgery is finished?"

Response: "Mrs. Hill, in some ways periodontal disease is like diabetes, but not quite as serious. I make this analogy only to explain to you that, just as diabetics are forever at risk when eating sweets, you have an increased risk of redeveloping periodontal problems. That is why it is even more critical that you pay careful attention to your home care habits and make regular professional maintenance appointments to help keep disease from redeveloping."

Keywords: diabetes, periodontal disease, regular dental cleanings

"PERIODONTAL TREATMENT"

Situation: This patient desires restorative and prosthodontic care, but a history of periodontal therapy has formed a block in his mind to repeating it.

Patient: "I don't want my gums cut on and scraped. I've had it done before. Just make me the crowns and bridge or partial and let's be done with it!"

Response: "Mr. Adams, one would never build a fine home on sandy soil without first developing the best of firm foundations. There is no way crowns and bridges will hold up to 200 pound chewing forces when attached to weak teeth. Your investment will serve you best by insuring it with sound periodontal therapy. Newer dental techniques with lasers and such have radically modified the way periodontal care is delivered for you."

Keywords: periodontal, foundation, re-treatment, new home, sandy soil

"PERIODONTAL TREATMENT"

Situation: This patient is tired of more needed treatments after extensive gum surgery and is balking at the time and expense involved in splinting periodontally-involved teeth.

Patient: "I still don't understand why you must bond my teeth together. I had a friend who had a retainer wire on the back of his teeth and he said it drove him crazy. Since the gum surgery fixed my gums, why can't we just leave it at that?"

Response: "Mr. Peterson, we need to splint your teeth together to give them better strength. Six single, shallow-rooted teeth are not as strong as one long six-rooted tooth, so to speak. Consider this analogy. If fence posts were not placed in deep-enough holes, they'd get loose in time. That is like your teeth's too-shallow roots are now. Anchoring them together, like bracing corner fence posts, strengthens them.

And, if the periodontally-treated teeth have a partial or bridge attached to them without being braced, it would be like hanging a heavy metal gate on a too-weakly-anchored fence post. It just wouldn't hold, and that would not be serving you properly."

Keywords: splinting, periodontal disease, expense

"PERIODONTAL TREATMENT"

Situation: This patient is unaware of growing periodontal problems, but is quite meticulous about her appearance, otherwise.

Patient: "Oh, my gums have always bled when I brush and floss them. They don't hurt. I guess it runs in the family."

Response: "Mrs. Vickers, bleeding from the gums is a sign of something wrong. For example, you can scrub healthy fingernails and cuticles vigorously without any pain or bleeding, even when using soap. But, try that with a hangnail or a cracked fingernail and it could bring tears to your eyes. The bleeding in your gums is the earliest sign that something is wrong. At this early stage, though, the gum disease is fairly easily corrected and recurrence prevented."

Keywords: bleeding gums, periodontal disease, cuticle, hangnail, hand scrubbing, pain

"PERIODONTAL TREATMENT"

Situation: This patient accuses her former dentist of failing to diagnose and/or inform her about a periodontal problem.

Patient: "Doctor, I have had my teeth cleaned every three months for years. My last dentist never said anything about gum disease. Now you are telling me that I have it? How long has this been going on? Why was I not told before?"

Response: "Mrs. Cobb, I appreciate your wonder. But, I can't speak into the past. Let me give you an analogy. If we both came up on an auto accident that had just occurred and a police officer came to us asking what had happened, we would have to answer that we didn't know. We had just gotten there. I don't know anything about your dental past, just what I see here now. The important thing is that we get started correcting it as soon as we can."

Keywords: periodontal disease, prior dentist

"PERIODONTAL TREATMENT'

Situation: The patient presents with heavy subgingival calculus and is suspicious of the diagnosis and/or the need for comprehensive root planing.

Patient: "You mentioned calculus, or tartar, on my teeth. I don't feel any. And, even if it is as bad as you say, I don't see why it takes four visits to get it all off. Everyone else I know just gets their teeth cleaned twice a year, with just one visit each time."

Response: "Mrs. Nelson, much of the calculus on your teeth is under the gum line. That's why you may not feel it. And it really grips the teeth well, like barnacles hooked onto a ship. You can imagine how much work it is to clean a ship's hull after years of buildup. Of course, your problem is not that severe. But, while barnacles just slow a ship down, calculus may cause a speeding up in the loss of your teeth. So, in another way it is even more serious. With the gums numb, the calculus can be safely removed. Since it is not as safe to numb your whole mouth at once, we choose to stagger the calculus

70

removal into two or four visits to make it easier on us both."

Keywords: barnacles, root planing, calculus, multiple visits

"PERIODONTAL TREATMENT"

Situation: The patient is inquisitive of the need for root planing, in spite of having had infrequent prophylaxes for years, as she detects no calculus herself.

Patient: "This calculus or tartar you keep talking about ... I guess I've been having my teeth cleaned off and on for years, although I've never really noticed calculus on them. Wouldn't I feel it?"

Response: "Mrs. Fleming, the fact that you have been having your teeth periodically cared for professionally is one of the reasons that you still have teeth today! Over the years, deeper calculus has developed under the gum line. This is a result of the hardening of the plaque that forms there if it is not completely removed every single day. Those shards of calculus under the gums are like pieces of broken glass, gouging the gums. Our special instruments sense the calculus. Now just happens to be that time when we must step in and meticulously remove it, tooth by tooth, and I just happen to be the dentist to have to tell you about your need for this."

Keywords: periodontal disease, shards   of glass, root planing, previous care

"PERIODONTAL TREATMENT"

Situation: This patient has periodontal disease, yet is not convinced of the need for gum treatments.

Patient: "But Doctor, my gums don't hurt and, besides, they've always bled. I really don't think I want to go through with any kind of gum treatment like you're talking about if I don't really need it."

Response: "Betty, I understand your apprehensions. Many kinds of problems can develop beyond repair before we know enough about them to begin action. Take termites, for example; an inspector may tell of an infestation, but you may reply that you've not seen any around, so you just wait. Six months later he tells you the same thing. You tell him you've seen one or two 'flying ants,' but that's not enough to worry about. Then, a year later he returns to tell you that floor joists are close to collapsing and that major reconstructive carpentry work PLUS expensive whole-house termite fogging is necessary. Gum disease usually doesn't hurt, but it is very destructive, nonetheless. Unfortunately, by the time it really does hurt, teeth are loosening and dentures are often the only option left."

Keywords: periodontal disease, termites, procrastination

"PERIODONTAL TREATMENT"

Situation: This young lady, at her first dental visit in six years, has been told that she needs four sessions of root planing. She is surprised at what the fee for her first "cleaning" in six years will be and is also in doubt about the need for two to four visits, since she has no pain from her gum disease.

Patient: "Doctor, the fee you quoted for my cleaning is more than ten times what Dr. Nextdoor charges. And, although it has been six years since my last cleaning, I can't believe dental fees have gone up that much!"

Response: "Mrs. Edwards, during the 6 years since your last dental visit, a lot of plaque and calculus has built up on your teeth. What has taken more than six years to form cannot be removed in one visit. Much of it is under the gum line and must be removed while your gums are numb. This is similar to an automobile problem. If, for example, your car's engine went too long without an oil change and began to act up, your quick oil-change center could not simply change the oil and everything be okay. In your case, your gums are bleeding, are tender to touch, and are swollen. They need more attention than what one visit can allow."

Keywords: root planing,automobile, periodontal, multiple visits

"PERIODONTAL TREATMENT'

Situation: This patient is unconvinced of having early periodontitis, owing to the absence of severe symptoms.

Patient: "My gums don't hurt at all. They just bleed a little when I brush my teeth. How can I have gum disease?"

Response: "Mr. Miller, let me make a comparison that I think will help you understand. Our chairs are sitting here on carpet. But, it's not like a hammock; the carpet is on firm flooring. We regularly vacuum our carpet, just as we should brush and floss our teeth. We have termite inspections for our home and we pay attention to leaky pipes. But, if the subflooring were to weaken due to termites or moisture, it could collapse. The gums and bone support your teeth, like the floor supports the carpet. Maintenance inadequacies can result in the loss of support."

Keywords: periodontal disease, flooring, support

"PERIODONTAL THERAPY"

Situation: This patient has difficulty comprehending what she has heard called a "deep cleaning."

Patient: "Dr. Gardner, why should I have this deep cleaning done if there's no pain? My teeth feel strong to me."

Response: "Mrs. Perkins, periodontal disease is a quiet disease. Just as you regularly vacuum your carpet, you regularly clean your teeth. When the condition of your rugs demands it, you call in carpet cleaning professionals. Right now, the roots of your teeth are very rough. I can predict with absolute certainty that they will become diseased. We have seen it too many times before. Until you've experienced meticulously-clean teeth and gums, you will not know what to appreciate."

Keywords: carpet-cleaning, root planing, rugs, vacuum periodontal disease

"PERIODONTAL DISEASE"

Situation: This young lady has gingivitis, yet seems to not be disturbed about it and has poor home care habits.

Patient: "Oh, doctor. My gums always bleed. Flossing makes them even worse. I'll just let you take care of them for me twice a year."

Response: "Jenny, I know you love roses. When you buy one from a nursery, it is removed from ideal growing conditions. Unless you maintain its needs, it will become diseased. Sure you can then spray it, but it will never be 'cured' – only to get sick again until you spray it again. Going through cycles of professional cleanings with repeated intermittent episodes of gum diseases is hard on your teeth. You must brush and floss your teeth every day; there's no question about it."

Keywords: roses, gingivitis, periodontal disease

"OCCLUSAL THERAPY"

Situation: This patient does not understand the need for having an equilibration performed before extensive reconstructive crown and bridge work is performed.

Patient: "If you are going to crown all of my teeth anyway, why do you have to adjust the bite beforehand?"

Response: "Mrs. Walker, it is like installing new linoleum flooring. If the floor below is not perfectly level, the new flooring will eventually settle — cracking and showing the irregularities below. A perfect foundation below guarantees the best possible result. The equilibration is like flattening out the floor in preparation for the new flooring."

Keywords: carpet, equilibration, linoleum flooring, unlevel floor

"OCCLUSAL THERAPY"

Situation: This patient does not want an equilibration, not understanding its true need and purpose.

Patient: "Doctor, why do you want to grind on my teeth? They don't feel out of sorts to me."

Response: "Mr. Hudson, our studies have concluded that your bite and teeth are out of balance. You know what an unbalanced car tire rides and steers like. If the tread on an unbalanced tire separates, it can cause an accident. Your jaw joints are the most complicated and sensitive joints in your body. Since they are out of balance, it is important to restore the harmony and prevent possible later damage."

Keywords: car tire, TMJ, equilibrate, balance

"OCCLUSAL THERAPY"

Situation: The patient resists occlusal adjustment following periodontal care, or even without it, in the presence of occlusal interferences and related mobilities.

Patient: "I really don't want my teeth ground on. I'm afraid they will get sensitive. Besides, they don't feel loose to me."

Response: "Mr. Craig, loose teeth are a lot like loose fence posts. When wiggled over time, like when cows rub on fences, the teeth get looser. Electric fences keep cows away. Since we can't put electric fences on your teeth, simple adjustments will better reinforce them for the chewing they perform each day."

Keywords: occlusal adjustments, bruxism, periodontal, mobility, electric fence

"OCCLUSAL THERAPY"

Situation: This patient will not accept having to have equilibration therapy accomplished before undergoing extensive reconstructive dentistry.

Patient: "I don't like the idea of having my teeth ground down. It'll make them even more sensitive than they are."

Response: "Mr. Carter, we selectively adjust the teeth until they all hit simultaneously. When you close, there are some places where they hit first. You can stand on a piece of glass laid on a perfectly flat floor without the glass breaking. But, put one small dry pea under it and that glass will break when stood on. If we place porcelain crowns in an uneven environment, they risk fracture from chewing forces because of bite errors placed on them. Maximum life for your dentistry demands an exact bite, attained by careful adjustment."

Keywords: equilibration, rehabilitation, glass

"OCCLUSAL THERAPY"

Situation: This patient cannot accept the need for occlusal therapy and needs an explanation to help crystallize the benefits in her mind.

Patient: "I don'tsee why my teeth need to be ground on or a splint made. They seem to mesh okay, even if they do slide around a lot."

Response: "I don't know if you have ever sat on a stool or at a table that has one leg shorter than the others, but you can imagine how annoying it is and how sore your leg could get trying to keep the chair or table propped from rocking. Similarly, your jaw muscles, as you may or may not have found, can get sore from 'propping' your teeth, so to speak. The splint we make for you is like temporarily shimming the short leg until we adjust everything."

Keywords: occlusal adjustment, equilibration, splint

"OCCLUSAL THERAPY"

Situation: This patient cannot understand the need to have an occlusal splint made, in light of the fact that teeth will need adjusting or restoring later, anyway.

Patient: "Why must we waste time with the splint when you are going to change my teeth later?"

Response: "Mr. Hall, the splint acts like air-leveling shock absorbers on an automobile. When you put a heavy load in the trunk, the shocks compensate by lifting the car and providing a smoother ride. We want to help give the teeth, muscles, and jaw joints a 'smoother ride.' Once we find the position that is most comfortable to you, we can reshape your teeth to that position for a permanent smooth ride."

Keywords: appliance, occlusal, splint, shock absorbers, restore

"OCCLUSAL THERAPY"

Situation: This patient resists occlusal splint therapy, even though he has morning head and jaw aches and opens his mouth widely only with some difficulty.

Patient: "Doctor. I don't see any need for a splint. I've had headaches since well before my jaw ever gave me trouble. Besides, my jaw doesn't bother me most of the day, anyway."

Response: "Jim, let's look at it this way. If you wore shoes that made your feet hurt, you might just blame the shoes, especially if your feet felt better when you had the shoes off. But, if you found shoes like Hush Puppies® that felt good all the time, wouldn't you want to wear them? That's what we would like to do with the splint, make your jaw feel comfortable all the time."

Keywords: occlusal, splint, shoes, comfortable, Hush Puppies®

"MAJOR RESTORATIVE DENTISTRY"

Situation: This patient wants to procrastinate about having crowns and onlays placed on endangered teeth.

Patient: "Why disturb them right now?

Nothing is bothering me. I'd rather wait until it really needs repairing: then, we can take care of it."

Response: "Mr. Dodd, it really DOES need restoring now. Your large fillings are wearing and the teeth are losing their support. Crowns protect them from uncontrollable fractures. It's a lot like riding on tread-worn tires. They are really close to blowing out, but you never know when that will be until it actually happens. No one knows how close these teeth are to failure. A crown will help protect that from happening."

Keywords: crowns, onlay, procrastination, tire blow-out

"MAJOR RESTORATIVE DENTISTRY"

Situation: This patient cannot understand the need to replace some restorations on teeth already slated for crowns.

Patient: "I don't see why you have to replace those fillings when you are going to crown those teeth in the first place."

Response: "Mrs. Moore, since those restorations were placed, anything could have happened underneath and to them. There may be cavities forming. They may have microfractures I cannot yet see. You know, there have been stories about Florida homes caving into sinkholes. If they knew those sinkholes were going to form where the homes were to be built, they would not have built them there, would they? Only restorations that give me doubt as to their ability to support crowns need replacing. Then, we can do the premium dental care you deserve."

Keywords: replace fillings, sink holes, fine home

"MAJOR RESTORATIVE DENTISTRY"

Situation: This patient has a difficult time understanding the need for the replacement of fillings before crown and bridgework is accomplished.

Patient: "If you are going to crown the teeth, why do you have to replace the fillings first? I thought x-rays were for seeing if there was decay under the old ones."

Response: "Mrs. Bradford, when all of the conditions are right, an artist creates a masterpiece. If that artist was forced to use notebook paper or newsprint, the work may not stand the test of time. These fillings were not initially intended to support crowns and bridges. But, they have served their purpose. Now we must insure that the beautiful dentistry you will receive will endure like a Rembrandt or Michelangelo creation."

Keywords: artist, painting, foundation, replacement of fillings, pre-treatment

"MAJOR RESTORATIVE DENTISTRY"

Situation: This elderly patient has been confronted with the need for extensive crown treatments.

Patient: "Doc, I am old, in case you haven't noticed. My teeth probably don't have but ten or fifteen years left, at best. I can't see the need for all of those crowns."

Response: "Mr. Abrams. I am sure you have noticed that as we get older our fingernails get more brittle. Well, so do our teeth; they thin from wear. In actuality, you may well live for twenty or thirty more years; no one ever knows. To make sure these teeth are still with you then, we must place the crowns to stop the chipping that is occurring."

Keywords: crowns, aging, brittle, fingernails

"MAJOR RESTORATIVE DENTISTRY"

Situation: The patient questions the need to keep a non-endangered tooth (teeth) that would need replacing on removal and is hesitant to invest in replacing teeth that are already missing.

Patient: "Doctor, even after you remove that tooth. I will still have 25 left. I eat fine with those, so one less won't hurt any, will it? And, as for replacing the ones that are already missing, this one too for that matter, I can't see where spending the thousands of dollars is worth it."

Response: "I appreciate your concern, Mr. Kelley. Let me make a simple analogy that I think will help make more sense of this. As you lose teeth, the others 'take up the slack,' so to speak. They have to work harder. If you were driving an eighteen-wheeled truck across the country and a tire blew out, you could remove the tire and continue with just seventeen wheels.

In time, though, the extra stresses would cause another to fail. Yet, you never know when it will happen. Your teeth are similar. They all work together and. as it is now, your teeth are like you're riding on less than eighteen wheels."

Keywords: truck driver, saving teeth, bridge, partial denture, tire blow-out

"MAJOR RESTORATIVE DENTISTRY"

Situation: This patient only wants the symptomatic tooth repaired, leaving others in need of treatment for later.

Patient: "I just want the one that's broken fixed. The others aren't bothering me yet."

Response: "Mr. Brooks, we could do that. But then, I would like for us to still be friends outside of this office. Your teeth all work together, like a football team does. Each player is important, whether the quarterback or the tackle. You know, it is essential that we fix that one tooth. Since all of your teeth work together as a team, it is actually more important that they be restored in harmony at the same time."

Keywords: football, team, symptomatic, procrastination

"CROWNS"

Situation: This patient is resistant to having a post and core (or buildup) and crown placed after a root canal is done.

Patient: "If the nerve is dead after the root canal, why crown it? Won't a filling do just as well?"

Response: "Mr. Lyle, the tooth will actually need both. Here's why. Just as a tree dies and becomes brittle, so does this tooth. Its internal life is gone. In time, a simple push by hand can topple that tree. Your tooth could succumb to something as soft as mashed potatoes. If it broke through the roots, no crown could save it. A crown now won't prevent it from becoming brittle, but it will help prevent cracking and breaking. The post and core (filling) is the foundation, insuring the proper support for the crown."

Keywords: crowns, dead tree, brittle, post-endo

"CROWNS'

Situation: This patient cannot accept the need for a crown, in spite of being aware of cracks in the teeth.

Patient: "If the crack is small, let's just leave it alone. It's barely noticeable and it doesn't cause me any complaint. We'll do the crown when I need it."

Response: "Mrs. Jones. I don't know if you have ever seen a badly cracked car wind-shield, but they can really look dramatic – running across the front, leaking, etc. And. in some states it is illegal to drive with them like that.

Now, it certainly isn't illegal to have a cracked tooth. That's your choice. My duty to you is to call it to your attention and let you know that if the crack radiates through the nerve or roots, the tooth may need to be removed and replaced, like a car's windshield. Only, this would require much more time on my part and yours and a lot more money as well, especially if a root canal was also needed. A crown placed on that tooth now will help prevent a broken tooth."

Keywords: cracks, windshield, replacement cost, crown

"CROWNS"

Situation: This patient is asking for temporary treatment until he can have a crown placed on a broken tooth.

Patient: "Well, I know I need a crown. I just can't afford it right now. Can you just get me by until I can get the crown?"

Response: "Well, Mr. Jordan, we can place a carefully constructed plastic filling buildup. If you are extremely careful with it, it should do okay and will act as the foundation for the crown later. You must not wait too long, though. It is like putting your household goods in a mini-storage building until you finish building a house. Time increases the chances of theft and mildew damage. In your case, the sooner you have the crown placed the less chance you will break the tooth so seriously that no dentist could save it."

Keywords: crown, buildup, mini-warehouse

"CROWNS"

Situation: This patient is uncertain of the need to crown an asymptomatic, cracked tooth which has not been extensively restored previously.

Patient: "I remember the dentist telling me that it would probably be the last filling that tooth would ever need. It's not that big, so how could the tooth be cracked?"

Response: "Mr. Smith, although that filling covers only the chewing surface, it still is big enough to act like a wedge. Much like we use wedges to split firewood, that filling has split your tooth, but thankfully not enough to warrant amputating it. A crown will hold it together and freeze the cracks where they are permanently."

Keywords: crown, cracked tooth, conservative, firewood, wedge

"CROWNS"

Situation: This patient is doubtful of the true need to have a tooth crowned.

Patient: "Do I really need this crown now?"

Response: "In a way. Mr. Frost, crowning a tooth is like buying insurance. You really don't know if you'll ever need it or not until it maybe is too late. If a tooth breaks through the nerve and roots, no amount of heroic dentistry may be able to save it. Even better than insurance, which helps pull your life back together in a crisis, a crown helps prevent a crisis."

Keywords: crowns, insurance, doubt

"CROWNS"

Situation: This patient wants a broken filling replaced and is rejecting a crown as he or she is not convinced of true need.

Patient: "I really don't see why a crown is needed. That filling lasted 15 years. Though it's cracked, it doesn't hurt. Can't you put another one in?"

Response: "I can understand how you feel. But a crown really is necessary. Here's an analogy. If you were having routine maintenance done for your car and the mechanic told you that your left front tire's tread was separating from the cord and could fail at any time, you wouldn't want to continue with it like that, would you? It's still holding air and rides okay, but you would still want the tire replaced because any extra miles would be unsafe miles. A cracked filling is equally unpredictable."

Keywords: crowns, flat tire, replacement filling

"CROWNS"

Situation: This patient is resistant to having an inevitable crown placed on a broken tooth and requests, instead, that another large buildup amalgam be placed.

Patient: "Can't we just patch this tooth up until it really needs that crown?"

Response: "Mr. Guy, patching it up is a lot like patching a leaking boat. The sad thing is that it gives out eventually. Even sadder is that, when it does, it's usually at an inopportune time. In a boat's case, it would be while in the water. In the tooth's case, it always seems while on vacation, a holiday, or during some other special function when you cannot see me right away. Then the real inconvenience starts. In addition, we never know how badly the tooth will break. If it breaks through the roots and the nerve, it can rarely be saved.

A little time and money invested in a crown now saves much anguish trying to make snap decisions later."

Keywords: crown, large amalgam, boat, on vacation

"CROWNS'

Situation: This patient does not understand the true purpose of a full-coverage crown.

Patient: "Doctor, give me one good reason why this tooth needs to be crowned."

Response: "Very simply put. John, if you had a broken arm you would definitely want it in a cast. Your tooth is cracked. Look at a crown for your tooth like a cast for your arm; only, the crown is never removed."

Keywords: crowns, cast, broken arm, permanent

"CROWNS'

Situation: This patient is flustered about having had a provisional crown come loose.

Patient: "For what I paid that temporary should hold up better than that, shouldn't it? It's aggravating to have to come back just to have it put back on."

Response: "Yes sir. I know it is a bother to come see us for such a short visit. But I appreciate your doing so. These temporary crowns are just that - temporary. They are a lot like space saver spare tires we see in newer cars these days. They aren't made for high speeds or high miles. While the temporary crown is quite durable, it does have its limits. If we put it on so tightly to insure it would adhere through anything, we would have quite a workout when it came time to place the permanent crown."

Keywords: temporary crown, provisional, coming off

"CROWNS"

Situation: This patient does not fully understand the need for preventive crowns over very large restorations.

Patient: "I really don't see the need for putting crowns on these teeth. The fillings are fine and the teeth aren't hurting."

Response: "Betty, in a way this is like being told by the mechanic changing your car's oil that your fan belt is worn and about to break. It would probably last a short while, but it would break eventually, probably in extreme heat. There would be serious problems like the engine overheating and becoming stranded on the road. The cost of taking a chance on the large fillings continuing to hold up, especially when they are used to eat popcorn, cherry pie, ice, or other hard foods, is likely to be greater than if we go ahead and place the crowns."

Keywords: crowns, uncertainty, fan belt, stranded

"CROWNS"

Situation: This patient resists crowns needed to definitively restore broken-down and extensively-restored teeth. She prefers to wait for breakage to occur before seeking definitive treatment.

Patient: "Yes. I can see cracks in my fillings (teeth). But, I think I'll just let you fix them when they do break. They've done okay, so far, all these years. I'll just eat soft foods."

Response: "Mrs. Jefferson, you've been lucky. Have you ever heard of an airplane that just lost an engine for no known reason? It may have had undetected hairline cracks. In any event, it's a shame that aircraft engines seem to fall off at the most inopportune time, when the plane is doing what it's supposed to be doing. Flying! Your teeth may do that; they may simply fail, and it usually occurs while eating. The sad thing is, it is usually at an inopportune time as well, like when on vacation, over the holidays, or on a Saturday night. And, if it is causing pain it may be an inconvenience for you if we can't get together immediately. The safe thing is to prevent that breakage and subsequent discomfort now."

Keywords: crowns, airplane engine failure, vacation, cracked teeth, cracked fillings, procrastination

"CROWNS"

Situation: This patient balks at having crowns made for his teeth. He prefers replacement fillings instead.

Patient: "Can't you just replace these broken fillings with new ones? I really can't afford to spend any more money than is necessary. Besides, I hear crowns cost over $500. Won't new fillings do me just as well?"

Response: "Mr. Black, each time we replace a filling it gets bigger. As it is, each is like a large wedge cutting the tooth in half. If you hit something just right it may drive the 'wedge' in. causing the tooth to crack, possibly even through the nerve. A crown will prevent that, capping the tooth much like farmers cover fence and gate posts with metal, protecting them from the elements."

Keywords: crown, large filling, expense, farm fence posts, wedge

"CROWNS"

Situation: This patient needs a crown for a broken tooth but insists on having a large, precariously-placed buildup performed instead.

Patient: "I'd rather you just fill it, Doctor. I hear crowns can cost over five hundred dollars. There is no way a filling will cost that much, is there?"

Response: "Mrs. Jackson, you wouldn't have much faith in an orthopedic surgeon who simply bandaged a badly-broken arm. You know a cast would be in your best interest and you would demand one. My placing an extremely large restoration in that tooth is similar. A crown is like a cast, only it is never removed."

Keywords: cast, bandage, broken arm, trust

"PROSTHETIC DENTISTRY"

Situation: This patient has severely worn anterior teeth due to missing posterior teeth.

Patient: "Doctor, why are my teeth worn so badly in the front? They didn't always look like this." (Or, you could bring this wear to your patient's attention using a mirror or study models.)

Response: "Mrs. Winter, the reason these teeth are worn so badly is because you are 'rabbit chewing.' Have you ever heard of this? A rabbit does not have back teeth to grind food so she has to use the front incisors. That's what you have to do. A rabbit's front teeth can continue to grow as they wear down. Unfortunately, your teeth won't grow any more. They just wear away. We must replace your missing back teeth to stop the wearing away."

Keywords: missing teeth, rabbit, rabbit chewing

"PROSTHETIC DENTISTRY"

Situation: The patient is apprehensive and discouraged about his new dental prosthesis. Over-expectancy has led to disillusionment.

Patient: "Doctor. I'm not sure I'll ever get used to my new dentures (partials). It feels like they are too big. And they don't feel solid, like real teeth."

Response: "Mr. Guy, you know they aren't real teeth. In fact, they are only 25% as effective, at best. The bulk you notice is the denture replacing teeth, bone, and the gums that are missing. Your tongue and cheeks have to get used to that again. When you first learned to walk you had to pay attention to each step. You fell, sometimes many times. But, you obviously got back up and soon were running. Over millions of Americans wear dentures or partials. They do fine and so will you, with time."

Keywords: first step, dentures, disillusionment

"PROSTHETIC DENTISTRY"

Situation: This patient has just received new dentures and she is overly-optimistic regarding their function.

Patient: "I can't wait to go out to dinner tonight. My husband is taking me out for steak so I can try out my new teeth. I've been waiting so long for this."

Response: "Go slow, Betty. Dentures function better than many other prosthetics like artificial arms and legs, but they are all alike in at least one way: you must 'ease' into them. Even then, they still aren't 100%. Just as you wouldn't attempt to run a race right after getting an artificial leg, you should never overwork your dentures. With an artificial leg, you would first learn to walk, then maybe work up to only a jog at best. You might never run a marathon because any prosthesis is still only the next best thing to real."

Keywords: dentures, over-expectant, prosthesis, artificial leg, run, marathon

"PROSTHETIC DENTISTRY"

Situation: This patient does not appreciate the true need to replace missing (or recently extracted) teeth.

Patient: "I don't see why we have to replace that tooth with a bridge (or partial). I still have some back teeth there to eat with, and I chew on the other side mostly anyway."

Response: "Mrs. Simpson, your teeth arc lined up like books on a shelf. If one is removed, the others next to it fall into that newly-formed space. Something similar begins the day a tooth is removed. Once it happens with a book, it's easy to replace the book. Not so with the tooth. Orthodontics, extractions, even TMJ therapy may be needed first. As you can see, all of that cannot be done as immediately and easily with your teeth as it can be with books!"

Keywords: missing teeth, books, prosthesis

"PROSTHETIC DENTISTRY"

Situation: This patient is "shopping" for dentures, with fee alone as the deciding factor. She is thinking about having them made at a dental lab through a denturist. The patient is allowing you the redemption of "meeting their prices" before she seeks treatment elsewhere.

Patient: "I want to have my dentures made at a denture lab. They can make a set for $450 complete. I'll be happy to let you make them, Dr. Goodman, if you can match their price."

Response: "I appreciate your concern with fees, Mrs. Jones. These days we all have to watch our money. Even though you may be able to obtain dentures elsewhere at a lower fee, often those dentures are not made under a dentist's prescription. Dentures must fit exactly to avoid irreversibly damaging the gums and, even worse, the bone. Put it in this perspective: you can put a piece of glass on a perfectly flat floor and walk on that piece of glass barefooted without breaking it. But, if you placed a single hard pea on the floor and laid that same piece of glass on top of the pea and then walked on it, that pea would act in a seesaw fashion and cause the glass to break. An exact fit with a denture is just one element of its success. The bite and many other factors involved are others. That's why a dentist must be involved in the denture prescription process."

Keywords: denturist, dentures, expense, fees

"PROSTHETIC DENTISTRY"

Situation: The patient is reluctant to leave her new dentures out of her mouth for a time each day to allow her gums to rest.

Patient: "Doctor, I don't see why I can't wear my new dentures all the time. I have for years. So has my husband. No one has ever told me before to leave them out."

Response: "Mrs. Overby, I am sharing with you the state-of-the-art thinking about denture use. You know, you don't leave your glasses on all the time because they may break when you sleep. We know to leave contact lenses out to rest the eyes. Dentures won't break leaving them in, but they can damage your mouth. Consider this example; if you've ever seen a spot on a green lawn where a board was left lying for some time, you know how the grass appears dead when you lift that board away. Lack of air and sunlight was bad for it. Your gums and the underlying bone must get some rest – preferably eight hours a day. Only you can decide when that will be and for how long. My duty is simply to share this information with you."

Keywords: denture, leaving out, gums, glasses, dead grass

"PROSTHETIC DENTISTRY"

Situation: This patient is uneasy about the "newness" of her dentures and is worried about getting used to them.

Patient: "Doctor, these new dentures fit well, but they don't feel the same as my old ones. I'm not sure I'm going to be able to get used to them. They feel bigger."

Response: "Mrs. Pryor, the reason your dentures feel different is because they are. They allow for all of the bone and gum changes that have taken place since your last ones were prescribed and compensate for them. You will get used to them in time. It's like driving a new or unfamiliar car. At first, you fumble for the light and wiper switches and the radio buttons. Soon, you are changing gears, adjusting the radio, and setting your cruise control all simultaneously! Your old dentures settled in. These will too."

Keywords: dentures, different, acclimation, new

"PROSTHETIC DENTISTRY"

Situation: Rather than take care of his remaining teeth, this patient would rather sacrifice them via extractions and either a full or partial denture.

Patient: "Doctor. I just want to let nature take its course, and when my teeth give out. I'll have dentures made."

Response: "Mr. Kimble, once your teeth are removed and the dentures are made, there is no turning back. You feel that, based on the state that your natural teeth are now in, dentures would be better for you. Restored to health, though, there's no substitute for your natural teeth. Everyone can't wear dentures for reasons like gagging. It is sad to find that out when it is too late. It's a lot like buying an expensive exercise machine and discovering that your knees just can't take it."

Keywords: exercise, gagging, dentures, extraction

"IMPLANTS"

Situation: This patient wants as few implants as possible to save money instead of an implant per tooth and wants bridges anchored to her natural teeth.

Patient: "Dr. Auger. I'd appreciate it if you'd attach the bridges to my teeth from the implants. Wouldn't that save me and you both trouble?"

Response: "Sandy, it would save you some money for now, but it would cause us both a lot of trouble. When you ride in a car the ride is smooth because of shock absorbers. When just one of them is broken, the ride becomes terrible! Asking a bridge to share an implant and a tooth both is like that analogy; since the tooth can give a little but the implant can't, the only thing that can really 'give' is the bridge itself."

Keywords: implants, anchoring, bridge, shock absorber

"ENDODONTIC THERAPY"

Situation: The patient is resistant to endodontic therapy, having heard from family and/or acquaintances that teeth treated by such tend to be lost anyway.

Patient: "Even if I have the root canal you say I need, what if I lose the tooth anyway? I've had people tell me they had to have their tooth pulled later after the root canal was done. What guarantee can you give me that it will work?"

Response: "Mr. Anton, root canal treatments work most of the time, with the few failures due to difficult tooth anatomy or really bad abscesses. Just as your Maker's dentistry comes without a warranty, can you really expect any better from me? Your attention to keeping needed appointments and good home care habits are what matters. If we both do our best, shouldn't we expect the best?"

Keywords: root canal, extraction, religious, best

"ENDODONTIC THERAPY"

Situation: This patient is having a difficult time understanding endodontic therapy.

Patient: "I still don't see why you have to fill the inside of the tooth if there will be a crown over the whole thing."

Response: "Mrs. Ford, look at the endodontic therapy as if it were the packing in a cardboard box. If you stood on an empty cardboard box, it would collapse. No empty cardboard box can support very much weight. But, if you packed the box full of books, we both could stand on it. Since the nerve in this tooth is dead and it is now hollow, it must be strengthened from within, much like putting the books within the box."

Keywords: endodontic therapy, cardboard box, books, strength

"ENDODONTIC THERAPY"

Situation: This patient cannot understand the intricacies of endodontic therapy.

Patient: "Doctor. I don't understand what a root canal is. I know people who have had it done, but it still sounds scary. Let's just pull this tooth."

Response: "Mr. Chapman, let me give you a simple analogy. Just as a hard Tootsie Pop® sucker has a soft center, so does the tooth. If the sucker's center melted, it would have nowhere to drain out. Your tooth has abscessed, like the sucker's center melting, and the abscess has leaked into the area around the root tip. That's why it hurts to chew on it: the root tip is as tender as a splinter in a finger. By replacing the tooth's center with a warm, soft rubber filling the abscess cannot re-form."

Keywords: Tootsie Pop®, abscess, splinter

"PRIMARY TEETH"

Situation: A young child (or the parent) needs reassurance him about the fillings needed.

Patient: "Doctor Bill, I've never had a filling in my (child's) teeth before. Will it hurt?"

Response: "Johnnie, you have a handsome smile, and your mom wants you to keep that handsome smile! We have already cleaned the sugar bugs off the outside of your teeth. A few teeth have some on the inside. I'll take care of them! We'll wash them out to help keep your teeth handsome! Our loud whistle (handpiece) scares the sugar bugs out. We will catch them with the straw vacuum cleaner when they jump out! If we can't scare them all, we'll 'bump' them out with our bumper (slow speed handpiece)! Then, we'll make a fancy star for the tooth! See, even I have stars! Is a silver star okay?"

Keywords: child, amalgams, explanation

"PRIMARY TEETH"

Situation: A parent is not sold on the need to preserve his child's primary dentition.

Patient: "I can't see spending that kind of money for steel crowns and root canals for just baby teeth. Since they are going to come out anyway, why can't we just pull them now so the permanent tooth can come on in?"

Response: "Mr. Ford, the baby teeth are like cars in a mall parking lot at Christmas. When a car pulls out of a space and is gone, someone else is going to hurry and take its place. If the permanent tooth is not yet ready to come in, then the adjacent baby teeth may shift, messing up the "parking lines' a bit. Eventually, permanent teeth may end up being 'parked' in the roof of the mouth or out toward the cheek, once the 'parking lines' are disregarded."

Keywords: expense, parking spaces, pulpotomy, stainless steel crowns

"NITROUS OXIDE"

Situation: This nervous patient is uncertain of the effectiveness of nitrous oxide.

Patient: "Dr. Pleasant, I'd really just like to be put to sleep. Can't you do that and get all of my treatments over with in one appointment?"

Response: "Ed, we would have to put you in the hospital for that. We have nitrous oxide here and it is very effective. If you will think back to childhood, riding in the back of the family car on a long, tiring trip, you might remember how pleasant it was to nod off during the ride. Nitrous oxide feels very, very much like that — pleasant. It has helped many apprehensive patients."

Keywords: nitrous oxide, nervous, long car rides

"EXTRACTIONS"

Situation: This patient, with a noncontributory past history of heart trouble, displays no interest in saving diseased teeth.

Patient: "Doctor, that tooth is probably too far gone to warrant investing good money in it. Let's remove the ones that need crowns and such and replace them all with a partial (or denture)."

Response: "Mr. Hudson, back when you had heart trouble, you trusted your doctor to correct your problems. He may have used a bypass operation or medicine — maybe both. But, he never considered an artificial mechanical heart because your own heart could still be saved. This tooth can be saved and to approach it from any other angle would be akin to malpractice, in my thinking."

Keywords: heart, bypass surgery, extraction

"EXTRACTIONS"

Situation: This patient is more interested in extractions than restorations, primarily from a cost savings standpoint.

Patient: "Doctor, I would rather you just pull this tooth instead of filling it. My fillings never last and fall out eventually anyway."

Response: "Mr. Reese, if you had an ingrown toenail you would not ask the doctor to amputate your toe! Your cavity is not hurting so badly that amputating the tooth is the only solution, is it? It really would be sad to amputate a tooth that could otherwise be re- sculpted with silver (bonding), just to save $50 or $100, wouldn't it?"

Keywords: extraction, expense, complacency, amputate

"EXTRACTIONS"

Situation: This patient has still-correctable dental problems, but has expressed plans for sequential extractions and dentures.

Patient: "I'd rather you just extract it, Doctor. When all is done, I will get dentures."

Response: "Mr. Wall, 12 of your teeth need attention. So, there are 12 possible episodes of pain like this one. If you are traveling it will be an inconvenience for you to be away from us seeking healing. Liken this to a car's transmission that people care for in two ways. They either have it serviced regularly, or they wait for a breakdown and invest in an overhaul. Once we get your dental needs caught up, inexpensive maintenance sessions can help prevent any needed major rehabilitation. As transmissions often fail when away from home, sadly, so do diseased teeth."

Keywords: dentures, extractions, transmission, traveling, maintenance care

"EXTRACTIONS"

Situation: This patient desires sequential extractions and the placement of complete dentures rather than undergo comprehensive restorative care.

Patient: "Doctor, rather than spend all of that money and time redoing my teeth, I think I would just rather have them all removed and get some dentures. That way, I will not have to worry about them anymore."

Response: "Mr. Rogers. I'm a member of the right-to-teeth movement. It is my obligation as a part of my profession's philosophy that I help you, in every way possible, to save your teeth. I must refuse to help extract all of your teeth. Because I wouldn't have it done to myself, I can't participate in it happening to you."

Keywords: dentures, restorative treatment, self

"WISDOM TEETH"

Situation: This patient has impacted wisdom teeth that need to be removed.

Patient: "Doctor, I have heard many bad things about having wisdom teeth removed. I think I will just wait until they start hurting to have anything done about them."

Response: "Mrs. Cleveland. I well understand your reluctance about having your impacted wisdom teeth removed. However, those teeth are like ticking time bombs that could go off at any time. You need to 'defuse* those bombs before you have trouble."

Keywords: wisdom teeth, time bomb

"HABIT APPLIANCE"

Situation: This patient is uncertain of a tongue thrust appliance for her child.

Patient: "I'm not crazy about having something in my child's mouth with prongs on it jabbing his tongue when he swallows."

Response: "I appreciate your concern, Mrs. Cox. It really is not as bad as it sounds. It is critical if we are going to get Billy's smile and teeth back in order. You know, a farmer sometimes has to use electric fences to keep cows from damaging fencing. This is truly different from that, just as Billy is certainly no cow! I make the comparison simply to point out that, like a cow's reflex to rub an itch on barbed wire, we all must swallow; that's a reflex too. Electric fences 'remind' cows not to go near the wire. This appliance just helps remind the tongue to go where it is supposed to when swallowing."

Keywords: tongue, electric fence, habit appliance

"SPECIALTY REFERRALS"

Situation: This young mother likes you and does not want her child sent to an orthodontist.

Patient: "I don't know, doctor. I'd really rather you take care of his crooked teeth. After all, Billy trusts you."

Response: "I like Billy too, Ms. Canady. Sometimes, though, certain needs should he met by someone with more practice. It is like building a house; a general contractor organizes what needs to be done and brings in plumbers, electricians, and the like to help him. It's not just to satisfy regulations; it makes for a better home. Legally, I could treat Billy, but I don't think it would be in anyone's best interest. I trust Dr. Straight and when you meet him, I believe you will see why."

Keywords: orthodontist, referral, specialist

"SPECIALTY REFERRALS"

Situation: This patient would rather a general dentist see about her child's orthodontic needs because it is less expensive and his office is closer.

Patient: "Dr. Goodman, I appreciate your caring for my kids. If you say that braces are needed, I trust you. I know my neighbor's dentist does braces too, and his office also cleans teeth and does fillings. I really do not like changing dentists just to have braces put on Billy's teeth. I like staying with one dentist. Is there anything wrong with switching our records to Dr. Nextbest so he can take care of all of our needs?"

Response: "Mrs. Joiner, I appreciate your confidence and I understand your concern. Dr. Nextbest is a good dentist. However, Billy's orthodontic needs really demand that a specialist treat them. That's why I have referred you to an orthodontist. You and your entire family are certainly still welcome here for your regular dental care needs. To give you an idea of why I would like Dr. Straight to see Billy for his braces, let me give you an analogy. If you had an old pickup truck that you just used to take trash to the landfill and it developed transmission troubles, you would probably just have the local auto repair 'shade-tree mechanic' fix it. But, if that vehicle was a car that you counted on for commuting to work and for carrying the kids on vacations, you would certainly want experienced hands caring for it. That is why there are specialty repair centers such as Aamco® transmission centers and others that perform mostly transmission work."

Keywords: orthodontics, expense, general dentist

"SPECIALTY REFERRALS"

Situation: A patient does not like being sent to a specialist for a dental procedure and would rather you, his or her general dentist, perform the procedure instead.

Patient: "Why can't you do this root canal (or extract this wisdom tooth) for me so I will not have to drive to an entirely different town to see a doctor I do not even know?"

Response: "Mrs. Henson, if you had to have heart surgery, even if you really like your family doctor you would not want him or her to do it, would you? We perform simpler root canals (extractions), much like your family practice physician treats mild heart disorders medicinally.

We always want you to have the best. That's why we would like a specialist to take care of it this time. If I were to treat this for you myself, the only advantage I can see is that I would get to keep the fee myself. That has never been my motivation and I will not start it now."

Keywords: endodontist, oral surgeon, specialist, referral

"SPECIALTY REFERRALS"

Situation: This patient is unhappy about being sent to see an endodontist. He trusts you and prefers your care to that of "a stranger."

Patient: "But Dr. Goodman, I really am not too happy about seeing a stranger; you've been my dentist for years. Can't you do this root canal?"

Response: "Ted, I sincerely appreciate your trust. Dr. Reamer is no stranger, though. I've known him for years. Just as movie directors coordinate camera operators and the actors, I coordinate ideal dentistry for you. I do some root canals, but the shape of the canals in your tooth requires extra skill and special instruments that I simply don't have. You can trust Dr. Reamer. I'll still be here to take care of you when you two finish working together."

Keywords: referral, endodontist, hesitant

"WAITING"

Situation: This patient is perturbed at her appointment running a bit late, affirming that she should be seen immediately.

Patient: "I'd like to know why doctors always run late. Why make an appointment in the first place? Maybe I should just start coming 30 minutes later."

Response: "Mrs. Poindexter, we are very sorry you had to wait. Sometimes the office can be likened to a classroom where a teacher has asked the children if anyone has a question. Naturally, several hands go up. Yet, the teacher, if she is a good one, answers each child individually, taking the time needed to do her job properly.

I know that is how you'd like your children treated. Here, though, we work very hard to keep things moving as best we can, but not at the expense of the quality of your dental care. Again, we are very sorry for your delay."

Keywords: wait, delays, teachers

"WAITING"

Situation: This young mother is impatient at having to wait to be summoned for her appointment. She is voicing her displeasure.

Patient: "I don't have time to wait around like this. I have to cook supper and do a million other things. Why do we always have to wait at doctor's offices?"

Response: "Mrs. Stevens, we are sorry for the delay. I guess a busy office is like a family with several kids. A mother wants to give her children the best, so she cares for each child one at a time: the quality of care is always most important. We must oversee every patient individually and we can never really predict exactly how long each visit will take. However, our team makes a wonderful attempt at keeping me on schedule without sacrificing the quality of care that everyone demands."

Keywords: wait, delays, motherhood, children

"DAYS OPEN"

Situation: This patient is asking about Saturday or evening appointments, times when you are not able to be open.

Patient: "I really want to come in on a Saturday morning or maybe a Tuesday evening after I get off work. Why don't you have anything on those days?"

Response: "Mr. Russell, doctors and team members can be likened to batteries, of which there are two kinds: regular and rechargeable. Rechargeable batteries can run down, but recharging makes them reliable again. Regular batteries might last a little longer, but when they expire, it is for good. We are like rechargeable batteries and we use evenings to recharge from each day and weekends to rest from our week."

Keywords: weekends, evenings, appointments, batteries

"DAYS OPEN"

Situation: This patient has asked about after-work appointment times, including evenings and Saturdays, of which you offer neither.

Patient: "I would really rather come in on a Saturday morning or after work one evening during the week. Why don't you have anything then?"

Response: "Mr. Bell, dentists' hours are not regulated like airline pilots' or truck drivers' hours, who are limited in how many hours they can fly or drive each month or day and use log books to document their schedules. We have to use a lot of care to be sure we don't overextend our doctor's time, since there are no legal constraints. This is just one of the ways we insure safe and quality care for our patients."

Keywords: hours, Saturdays, evenings, appointments, airline pilots, truck drivers

"HOME CARE"

Situation: This teenager is unmotivated about brushing and flossing.

Patient: "Dr. Pullman, no one else flosses. Why should I? Besides, I'm too busy hanging out."

Response: "Joey, I don't know if you've ever thought about it, but seeing how you are now old enough to go out with girls, you might want to pay special attention to your teeth — and your breath. I remember one young lady told me that kissing some guys is like licking an ashtray. You don't want to be talked about like that, do you?!?"

Keywords: ashtray, teenager, home care, kissing

"HOME CARE"

Situation: This pet lover seems to care for her animals more than her own mouth!

Patient: "I don't know, doctor... I don't have time to floss every day. It seems like they're getting so many cavities that I'll lose them all anyway. What's the use?"

Response: "Stephanie, we know that with proper care your teeth will last you forever. We know that pets live longer than wild animals because we give them the best of care. The same is true for our teeth; in the best conditions – daily brushing and flossing and regular checkups, they can be expected to last you a lifetime. We believe that because we see it every day! You will too if you do your part!"

Keywords: pets, flossing, brushing

"HOME CARE"

Situation: This youngster argues that flossing hurts.

Patient: "Dr. Stringer, it hurts when I floss. I brush every day; isn't that enough?"

Response: "Bobbie, brushing just cleans half of your teeth — the outside and inside halves. It doesn't touch the in-betweens. Flossing does. It's like being barefoot at the beach. The first day or two it's hot on your feet. Your feet quickly acclimate and your tolerance improves. Flossing is just like that. Sure, it's not as fun as going to the beach, but it really is more important."

Keywords: beach, flossing, bare feet

"HOME CARE"

Situation: This patient dislikes flossing because of initial gingival discomfort and has stopped flossing because of the gingival soreness.

Patient: "Flossing made my teeth and gums real sensitive. I did it for a while, but then I stopped."

Response: "Like exercise, flossing may cause soreness for a short while when you first start. But then, your gums become firm, like the muscles do, and things get better."

Keywords: flossing, soreness, exercise, firming up

HOME CARE"

Situation: This patient is not sold on flossing, and it is difficult to convince her of its importance.

Patient: "Doctor, I don't have any problems brushing my teeth. It's the flossing I just cannot get into. Can't my toothbrush alone do the job?"

Response: "Mrs. Crawford, when you wax a large dining room table or vacuum a carpet, you do the entire surface. If only half cleaned, the adjacent uncleaned surface looks even worse. If you considered each tooth in your mouth as a box, the toothbrush can clean the front and back surfaces fine. It's in-between that gets missed. Only floss can get in there. Without that, the spaces become yellowed, decayed, get diseased, and then stand out noticeably."

Keywords: flossing, vacuuming, half-done

"HOME CARE"

Situation: This patient is not yet sold on daily flossing and brushing; she is very busy and owns a home-cleaning business.

Patient: "Doctor, there's just no time for me anymore. Thankfully I have you twice a year! I floss when I can."

Response: "Jessie, I know you are proud of your cleaning business. I am sure that you appreciate why it is so important to prevent mildew in showers. Once it's there, it's difficult for the customer to permanently remove it on her own without your professional help.

Simply wiping the tile dry after each shower prevents the mildew, doesn't it? It's not much different with your teeth and dental disease. That's why I'd like you to floss your teeth once a day!"

Keywords: flossing, mildew, tile, brushing

"HOME CARE"

Situation: This patient cannot find the time to floss her teeth every day, although she is a good brusher.

Patient: "I just don't have the time to clean my teeth the way you're telling me I have to do!"

Response: "Yes, we live in a hectic world. You know, it takes a fair amount of time to wash your hair, doesn't it? You must blow it dry and style it. But, it's a known fact that people notice a smile before hair. Three minutes, twice a day, is truly all it takes to maintain a healthy smile by flossing and brushing. It may take a little more time at first as you get used to it again, but just as you wash, dry, and style your hair without much thought, you will also develop a routine for cleaning your teeth."

Keywords: flossing, brushing, time constraints, hair care

"HOME CARE"

Situation: This patient cannot be convinced to use a soft toothbrush, insisting on hard or medium bristles that "clean better."

Patient: "You tell me to use a soft toothbrush, but it doesn't clean my teeth as well as a hard one. They don't feel as good."

Response: "Mrs. Lumpkin, the best way to explain why a soft bristled brush really does clean better than a hard one is to give you an example that I think will help you better understand. Have you ever had to sweep spilled sugar or salt up off the floor? If you have ever tried it with a straw broom, you know how difficult it is to get it all into the dustpan. But, if you've ever used a broom with fine edges, you know how effectively that broom cleans. Another example is if you were to try and shine your shoes with a hairbrush. You know it would never work. But think how bright and shiny the lightest strokes with a camel-haired brush get your shoes. Toothbrushes are no different; the hard ones scratch and the soft ones polish."

Keywords: toothbrush, soft, hard, shining shoes, sweeping spilled sugar, bristles

"TOOTHBRUSH ABRASION"

Situation: This patient has abraded the gingival third of some of her teeth from overly-aggressive tooth brushing, making some teeth sensitive, and needs a clearer mental image of how it happened.

Patient: "I don't understand how a nice, soft toothbrush can make my teeth sensitive. I thought brushing was good for my teeth and gums. Now I don't know what to do."

Response: "Mrs. Taylor, toothbrush cuts can happen by using any kind of toothbrush, soft, medium, or hard. Abrasive toothpastes can enhance the effect. It's like this comparison: If you take the same path across a green grass lawn several times a day, eventually a trough will be worn through it. This is similar to what has happened to your teeth. Constant side-to-side brushing has ditched them out at the gum line, one of the most vulnerable places. It can make them very sensitive, since the distance to the nerve is shorter. Over time, the cuts can get quite deep. Remember, the Grand Canyon, as tremendous as it is, was formed simply by water and time. Let me show you a better way to brush along the gum line."

Keywords: toothbrush cut, erosion, cervical abrasion, Grand Canyon, path in grass

"FLUORIDE"

Situation: This patient is unsure of the benefits of topical fluoride, weighing the expense of the treatment.

Patient: "Doctor... I don't know if I'll have the fluoride today. Money's tight, you know. Can't I do without it?"

Response: "Terry, I'm sure you've heard of Teflon®-like car engine additives some auto mechanics recommend that really cut friction and make engines last longer. With your teeth freshly polished of everything foreign, now is the time to coat them with a super-strong barrier of fluoride. It's the next-best thing to Teflon® for your teeth."

Keywords: fluoride. Slick 50®, hesitant, cost

"PRESCRIPTIONS"

Situation: This patient is reluctant to spend money on an antibiotic prescription for a dental infection, or has an aversion to taking medicines.

Patient: "Doctor, I will hang on to this prescription and if the infection gets bad enough, I'll get it filled."

Response: "Mr. Lee, that is dangerous. Here is why; any infection in your head, just inches from your brain, needs treating. You know, a small brick propped behind a single tire of a truck will keep the truck from rolling down an incline. But not even several of those bricks will stop the truck if it begins rolling before that single brick can be placed there. These antibiotics keep the infection from getting away from us, which could require hospitalization and maybe even IV drug administration."

Keywords: antibiotics, reluctance, wheel chock, truck, hospitalization, brain infection

"SEALANTS"

Situation: A young mother needs a simple description about bonding or sealants to help calm her child's (and/or her) fears.

Patient: "Doctor, could you please explain how you are going to put those sealants on her teeth?"

Response: "Sure. Bonding to teeth is a lot like putting polish on your fingernails. You wash the surface, paint it on, and then let it dry. One of the differences here is that we use a special light to speed up the drying process. You see, it's really very, very simple."

Keywords: sealants, fingernail polish, child

"TREATMENT PLAN CHANGE"

Situation: In the course of treatments, a planned procedure is discovered to no longer be possible, necessitating a revamping of the original treatment plan.

Patient: "If you thought this could happen, why didn't you plan for it in the first place? Now we have to start all over."

Response: "I really am sorry. Mrs. Frost. I could go through with our plans, but the result would never make you or me happy. This is akin to restoring a fine antique sofa. Only after removing the fabric can we evaluate the frame and springs to be sure they are suitable for covering with the new cotton and fabric. But, being it is so valuable, it is worth the little extra effort and expense to save a one-of-a-kind."

Keywords: change, antique, treatment plan

"TREATMENT PLAN CHANGE"

Situation: This patient has just been told of the need to change the treatment plan because of unforeseen findings.

Patient: "I thought we had it all planned. Now we have to start over? Can't we just stick to the plan, since I have so much time and money invested?"

Response: "Mrs. King. I am sorry for the change. It would not be in your best interest to pursue our original plans. It is like taking your mother's or grandmother's heirloom wedding gown in to be cleaned in preparation for another wedding. If the dry cleaner recommended replacing the weak panels before continuing, you would acquiesce, otherwise the bride would not be very happy come the wedding day. I simply want you to be happy with me and what I have done for you."

Keywords: wedding gown, dry cleaning, repair, change, treatment plan

"DENTURE ADJUSTMENTS"

Situation: This patient is becoming impatient with her denture adjustments.

Patient: "I don't know why it is taking so many visits to get these to fit right. My first set fit perfectly the first day. I don't know if I can stand too many more trips down here."

Response: "Mrs. Preston, I am sorry it is taking a few additional visits to reach the level of perfection that I demand. But remember, these dentures are fine instruments, just like a new grand piano. Once it is delivered it takes a return trip or two to finish the fine tuning. Soon, your dentures will be 'tuned.' so to speak, and will work for you as beautifully as music from the piano!"

Keywords: piano, tuning, dentures, adjustments

"FILLING ADJUSTMENT"

Situation: This distinguished gentleman is upset at having to "waste time" coming back to have a filling adjusted.

Patient: "Considering everything that went into doing this filling, I'd have expected it to be right the first time."

Response: "Mr. Phelps, we appreciate your appreciation! That filling took effort. Unfortunately, you were numb yesterday and couldn't tell us where to adjust it then. Believe it or not, it is only off by the width of a grain of sand. Like a very small pebble in a shoe, though, it is quite noticeable. And, just as with the pebble, it is equally easy to remedy!"

Keywords: adjustment, filling, pebble, shoe, grain of sand

"FILLING ADJUSTMENT'

Situation: This gentleman has had to return to have a high spot adjusted on a large restoration or a crown. In light of the initial expense, he is not very understanding.

Patient: "When you pay that much for something you expect it to be right. I can't see why everything wasn't tended to when I was here last time."

Response: "Mr. Peabody, I am sorry it is taking an extra visit to reach the level of perfection that the body demands. But please remember, this restoration (crown) is a fine instrument, just like a new grand piano. Once it is delivered it may take a return trip to finish the tuning. Soon, your restoration (crown) will be 'tuned,' so to speak, and will work for you as beautifully as music from a grand piano!"

Keywords: adjustment, high spot, crown, filling, restoration, piano, music

"REGULAR DENTAL CARE"

Situation: This young patient must be sold on the importance of regular preventive dental visits.

Patient: "I don't see the need for coming in twice a year. If I skip a visit or two, will that much more tartar be there? Besides, it costs a lot of money to have your teeth cleaned twice a year!"

Response: "Mrs. Tate, regular dental care is kind of like gardening. If you casually pull whatever weeds you see each week, the job is simple and uneventful. However, if you let four or five months pass, that weeding job is a real chore. If you let it go for years, the flowers will all be gone and the weeds will dominate. Your regular dental visits actually save you money and time in the long run, like regular and frequent weeding of the garden."

Keywords: regular care, weeding, garden

"STUDY MODELS"

Situation: This young apprehensive child needs a soothing explanation of the impression process.

Patient: "Dr. Goodman, I don't think I am going to like having those stone models made. Can't we do without them?"

Response: "Amy, we want to have a copy of your teeth just as they are right now, much like a monument or statue. The putty Jenny will mix and have you bite into is very much like pudding. The bad part is you don't get to swallow it, since we need all that we can to make the statues of your teeth!"

Keywords: alginate, impression, child, models

"PRIOR DOCTOR"

Situation: This patient claims her last doctor did not identify the problem you have just diagnosed, even though he has been seeing him regularly.

Patient: "Dr. Mizdit never talked about periodontal disease (crowns, etc). It seems to me that he would have urged me to have that done if it was really necessary. Why didn't he say anything about all of this?"

Response: "Mr. Roundtree, I cannot answer that. All I can say is that I am like the referee in a basketball game. I call it as I see it. That is judgment – one of the things you are paying me for. The most important thing is that we get to work correcting your problem right away."

Keywords: prior dentist, failure to diagnose, basketball, referee

"APPOINTMENTS"

Situation: This patient is mildly upset at having to wait two weeks to be seen for a minor dental reparative procedure.

Patient: "I don't see why it takes two weeks to get an appointment for such a simple filling. Can't you just work me in between patients today? Why does it always have to be 'we can see you in two weeks?'"

Response: "Mrs. Blackstone, if we thought that tooth was going to cause you an inconvenience before your appointment day, we would take care of it today. I really am sorry for the delay. (This can be added, with a smile, in responding to a patient who can be humored.) Look at it this way. If a movie is a really good one, the ticket line is always longer, isn't it?"

Keywords: appointment, delays, good movie

"BUSY OFFICE"

Situation: This gentleman insists on an unreasonably timely appointment in your busy, traditional solo-practice, questioning your unavailability of evening hours.

Patient: "I don't see why you can't see me when I get off work at 5:30 Wednesday. Other doctors see patients then."

Response: "Yes sir, some do. But we work hard to not just take care of patients but our team members as well. You know, in major league baseball there is a rule that a pitcher must rest between games. Otherwise, managers might abuse the good ones and schedule them too often, which would hurt their careers. We help as many patients as we can while remembering to replenish ourselves. After all, dentistry really is the 'big leagues,' isn't it?"

Keywords: baseball, busy practice, waiting

"COTTON ROLLS/GAUZE"

Situation: This young child is anxious to know about everything that is happening. Even the cotton rolls alarm her.

Patient: "I don't want all of that stuffed in my mouth. I won't be able to talk!"

Response: "Cindy, we're just going to put a few soft cotton rolls where we want it to stay dry, almost like a diaper for your teeth!"

Keywords: cotton roll, diaper, child

"RETRACTION CORD"

Situation: This patient requires constant explanation about what is going on to help keep her calm. Naturally, everything must be shared in laymen's terminology.

Patient: "What is that string you're putting around the tooth? Does that help hold the temporary crown in?"

Response: "No, Allyson. It is a special soft string that we gently place around the tooth, like a necklace goes around your neck. It pushes the gums back temporarily so we can make an ideal impression for your crown. It works much like when you push your cuticles back in manicuring them."

Keywords: retraction cord, crowns, necklace, manicure, cuticle

Made in the USA
Coppell, TX
02 November 2023

23737478R00100